Low-GI Weight Loss Made Simple

A Step-by-Step Glycemic Index and Load Guide with Food Swaps, Meal Plan & Recipes

mf

Disclaimer

This guide is provided for informational and educational purposes only and should not be interpreted as medical, nutritional, or professional advice. The author is not a licensed physician, nurse, dietitian, or mental health provider. Reading this guide does not establish a patient–provider relationship of any kind.

Always seek the guidance of a qualified healthcare professional before starting, changing, or discontinuing any supplement, diet, or lifestyle program. If you are pregnant, breastfeeding, managing a chronic medical condition, or taking prescription medications, consult your physician or pharmacist before considering any product mentioned in this guide.

The author and publisher make no representations or warranties regarding accuracy, applicability, fitness, or completeness of the information contained herein. While every effort has been made to ensure scientific accuracy and currency, medical knowledge and research evolve continually. Readers are responsible for verifying information and making decisions in consultation with licensed professionals.

Use of this guide and any information contained within it is at your own risk. The author and publisher disclaim all liability for any loss, injury, or adverse outcome that may result from the use or misuse of this material.

No supplement, diet, or practice discussed in this text is intended to diagnose, treat, cure, or prevent any disease. No outcomes or benefits are guaranteed.

Product names, supplement formulations, diet frameworks, and trademarks mentioned are the property of their respective owners and are used for identification only. Any images or illustrations that appear in related materials are licensed stock or educational placeholders.

Table of Contents

Introduction

Many people begin weight loss with optimism but quickly become frustrated by unstable energy, unexplained plateaus, and confusion about what to eat. These challenges are common in our modern food environment, where high-glycemic index (GI) choices such as white bread, sugary cereals, and processed snacks are everywhere.

Eating high-GI foods starts a cycle of rapid energy spikes and crashes. After consuming quickly absorbed carbs, blood sugar rises sharply and then drops, causing renewed hunger and cravings for more fast carbs. This cycle makes it hard to consistently reduce calories and maintain progress, as your body's signals become unreliable. Dieters often end up stuck, struggling with cravings and plateaus even when they believe they are "eating less".

This guide aims to cut through the confusion and provide straightforward answers. It does not focus on advanced blood sugar management, athletic carb cycling, or trendy supplements. Instead, it delivers evidence-based, practical steps to understanding glycemic index (GI) and glycemic load

(GL), the key principles that let you make informed, sustainable food choices. Mastering these concepts allows you to minimize blood sugar swings, feel satisfied, and achieve lasting weight loss.

The glycemic index ranks carbohydrate-containing foods by how quickly they raise blood sugar relative to pure glucose. Glycemic load goes further by accounting for the number of carbohydrates per serving. These tools let you see beyond simple calorie counts and better predict how meals will affect your appetite and metabolism. Learning to recognize high- and low-GI foods empowers you to plan meals, snacks, and restaurant choices more effectively giving you more control over hunger and progress.

This guide will teach you how to put GI and GL into practice in your daily routine. Upcoming chapters break down each step:

- You'll learn to read GI and GL charts, quickly gauging how foods affect blood sugar.
- Practical advice will show you how to assemble meals and swap high-GI foods for tastier low-GI options.
- Core meal planning tips will help you create a menu that supports weight loss, while batch-cooking and shopping ideas make it simple and affordable to stay on course.
- Every recipe and menu is designed to maximize satisfaction and steady energy, helping to avoid plateaus and reduce the urge to return to old eating habits.

- Troubleshooting tips and tracking tools will help you adjust, overcome setbacks, and monitor real progress.

If you're new or looking for a clear plan after previous trial and error, this guide focuses on practical steps and lasting results. A low-GI approach is not about strict limitation, but about steady, satisfying change that fits real life.

We'll start by exploring the science behind GI and GL, then guide you step by step in building meals, routines, and habits that eliminate dietary guesswork, support your weight loss goals, and help you feel your best every day.

Fundamentals of Glycemic Index and Load

Understanding the glycemic index (GI) and glycemic load (GL) is fundamental to achieving effective, sustainable weight loss through nutrition. These concepts allow you to see how your food choices directly impact your blood sugar and hunger, providing a science-based method to plan meals, shop smart, and avoid common dietary pitfalls. In this chapter, we'll break down what GI and GL are, show you how to use them in everyday decisions, and offer practical tools to help you make lasting changes.

What Are Glycemic Index and Glycemic Load?

The ***glycemic index*** is a ranking system for carbohydrate-containing foods. It measures how quickly and how much a food raises blood sugar levels after being eaten, compared to pure glucose, which is assigned a GI value of 100. Foods with a high GI are digested rapidly and cause a sharp spike in blood sugar, while foods with a low GI are broken down more slowly, leading to a gradual, smaller increase.

Glycemic load goes a step further by considering not just the quality (GI) but also the quantity of carbohydrates in a standard serving. This gives a more accurate picture of a food's actual impact on blood sugar. The formula for glycemic load is:

Glycemic Load (GL) = (GI × Net Carbs per serving in grams) ÷ 100

Net carbs are calculated by subtracting fiber from total carbohydrates, as fiber does not affect blood sugar the same way as digestible carbs.

Why Do GI and GL Matter for Weight Loss?

GI and GL are powerful tools for weight loss because they help you understand which foods will keep you full and energized versus those that may leave you hungry or craving more. Low-GI and low-GL foods support steady blood sugar, which reduces spikes in insulin, a hormone that both stores fat and triggers hunger when levels drop rapidly. By focusing on these foods, you can better control appetite and make it easier to maintain a calorie deficit without constant cravings.

Examples: How GI and GL Affect Your Meals

Let's look at how the GI and GL of different foods can affect your blood sugar and satiety:

- A ***white bagel*** (GI ~72) is made from refined flour and has a high carbohydrate content, resulting in a high GL and a rapid spike in blood sugar.
- An ***apple*** (GI ~36), despite its natural sugars, contains fewer digestible carbs per serving, giving it a low GL and a much milder effect on blood sugar.
- ***Lentils*** (GI ~32) are low in both GI and GL, providing energy gradually and supporting longer-lasting fullness.

These differences are essential when planning meals for weight loss and satiety. Choosing foods with a lower GI and GL can make a significant difference in how satisfied you feel after eating and how quickly you become hungry again.

Table 1: Sample Glycemic Index and Load Table

Food (Standard Portion)	Glycemic Index (GI)	Glycemic Load (GL)
White bread (1 slice, 30 g)	70	10
Rolled oats (½ cup cooked, 120 g)	55	13
Brown rice (½ cup cooked, 100 g)	50	12 (actual values may vary by source)
Chickpeas (½ cup cooked, 80 g)	28	8
Banana (1 small, 100 g)	51	13
Potato, boiled (1 medium, 150 g)	78	18
Lentils (½ cup cooked, 99 g)	32	7

Hundreds more values can be found in detailed charts available from reputable nutrition sources and appendices of many guides. Getting to know the GI and GL of your staple foods is a simple and effective way to control blood sugar and appetite.

How to Calculate Glycemic Load Using Food Labels

Calculating a food's glycemic load (GL) helps you estimate how much that food will affect blood sugar in a typical serving. Here's a simple step-by-step method:

1. ***Find the food's Glycemic Index (GI).***

   Look up the GI value in a reliable GI table or database. GI measures how quickly a carbohydrate-containing food raises blood sugar.

2. ***Check the net (digestible) carbs per serving.***

   On the nutrition label, find the ***total carbohydrates*** and subtract ***fiber*** to get net carbs.

   Net carbs = Total carbs − Fiber

3. ***Use the GL formula.***

   GL = (GI × Net carbs per serving in grams) ÷ 100

Example: Cooked Quinoa

- ***GI***: ~53
- ***Serving size***: ½ cup cooked
- ***Total carbs***: 20 g
- ***Fiber***: 2 g

- ***Net carbs***: 20 − 2 = 18 g

  $GL = (53 \times 18) \div 100 = 9.5$

So, a ½-cup serving of cooked quinoa has an estimated glycemic load of about 9–10, which falls in the low GL range.

Quick GL guide per serving:

- Low: 10 or less
- Medium: 11–19
- High: 20 or more

Using GL alongside portion size can help you choose carbohydrate foods that support steadier blood sugar levels.

This moderate GL suggests quinoa raises blood sugar less sharply than white rice or instant oats.

If you're dealing with a packaged food and can't find its exact GI, use the GI of the main carbohydrate ingredient. For example, for an oat bar, use the GI of rolled oats. If the product has added sugars or refined flour, the GI may be higher.

Glycemic Index Categories by Serving Size

GI values can be grouped as follows (by standard serving):

Low-GI: 55 or less

Moderate-GI: 56–69

High-GI: 70 or higher

Examples of Low-GI Foods (≤55):

- ***Lentils (½ cup cooked)***: GI ~32
- ***Sweet potato (baked, ½ cup)***: GI ~44
- ***Apple (1 medium)***: GI ~36
- ***Pear (1 medium)***: GI ~38
- ***Non-starchy vegetables***: GI 15–30 per cup
- ***Barley (½ cup cooked)***: GI ~28 (may vary by preparation method)

Moderate-GI Foods (56–69):

- ***Brown rice (½ cup cooked)***: GI ~50 (can vary by preparation method and rice type)
- ***Rolled oats (½ cup cooked)***: GI ~55
- ***Pineapple (½ cup)***: GI ~59
- ***Couscous (½ cup cooked)***: GI ~65

High-GI Foods (≥70):

- ***White bread (1 slice)***: GI ~70
- ***White rice (½ cup cooked)***: GI ~73
- ***Instant potatoes (½ cup)***: GI ~78 (estimate; check brand specifics)
- ***Watermelon (1 cup diced)***: GI ~76
- ***Cornflakes (1 cup)***: GI ~81

It's important to note that while the GI for a specific amount of food is fixed, eating larger portions will proportionally increase the glycemic load and the blood sugar impact.

Satiety, Blood Sugar, and Metabolic Effects

One of the most practical benefits of understanding GI and GL is in managing satiety and blood sugar swings. Here's how different food types compare:

- ***Low-GI foods***: These cause a slow, steady rise in blood sugar, helping you stay fuller for longer. Examples include oats, beans, lentils, non-starchy vegetables, and most whole fruits (not juice).
- ***Moderate-GI foods***: Useful as meal bases, especially when combined with protein or fiber. Examples are brown rice, rolled oats, and some tropical fruits.
- ***High-GI foods***: These trigger rapid spikes and subsequent drops in blood sugar, which can lead to increased hunger, cravings, and overeating. White bread, crackers, instant potatoes, and sugary cereals fall into this category.

A Quick Guide for Everyday Choices

- ***For steady energy and fullness***: Choose low-GI, low-GL foods and add protein and healthy fats.
- ***For stable blood sugar***: Combine moderate-GI foods with lots of vegetables, legumes, and protein.

- ***To reduce cravings***: Avoid high-GI foods, especially when eating alone or without protein and fiber.

If you find yourself feeling hungry soon after a meal, check whether the meal was based on high-GI foods or if it was lacking in fiber or protein. Adjust future meals accordingly to promote longer-lasting satiety and prevent unnecessary snacking.

Common Pitfalls: The GI/GL "Red Flag" Checklist

Even with the best intentions, it's easy to make mistakes that undermine your progress. Here are common pitfalls to avoid:

1. ***Believing all "whole grain" products are low-GI***: Many are made with finely milled flour and have a GI similar to white flour products.
2. ***Ignoring serving sizes***: GI is based on standard portions, but eating more increases the GL and the impact on blood sugar.
3. ***Choosing fruit juices or dried fruits over whole fruits***: These are often high-GI and sugar-dense, lacking the fiber found in whole fruit.
4. ***Eating sweetened cereals and instant grains***: Even those with added fiber or protein can have high GI/GL if they contain refined grains or sugars.

5. ***Picking "low-fat" snacks***: These often substitute sugars or refined carbs for fat, raising both GI/GL and reducing satiety.
6. ***Skipping protein or healthy fats***: Eating carbs alone can spike blood sugar and lead to quicker hunger; include protein and/or healthy fats to balance meals.
7. ***Misjudging starchy vegetables***: Potatoes, corn, and parsnips are higher-GI; consider leafy greens, broccoli, and peppers to keep GI/GL lower.
8. ***Trusting restaurant and convenience foods***: Sauces, coatings, and even "healthy" entrees can hide fast carbs that raise GI/GL.
9. ***Reducing fiber***: Skipping fruit skins, choosing white rice, or eating refined snacks removes fiber's moderating effect, causing sharper blood sugar spikes.

If your weight loss progress stalls, revisit this checklist. Small, repeated mistakes can add up and impact both your success and how full you feel after meals.

Moving from Fundamentals to Daily Practice

Now that you have a clearer understanding of GI and GL, along with sample charts, a calculation formula, food category tables, and a red flag checklist, you are equipped to start integrating these concepts into your daily routine. Whether you're planning oatmeal with berries, a chickpea salad, sautéed greens with lentils, or an apple as a snack, remember how small adjustments can yield significant results.

Here's how to put it into practice:

- Use the calculation steps for any new foods or packaged products you encounter.
- Check the food tables and red flags list when choosing between similar products or identifying trouble spots in your diet.
- Experiment with swapping high-GI grains for lower-GI options and notice how your energy and hunger respond.
- Prioritize whole foods, increase your intake of legumes, and pair carbohydrates with protein and healthy fats.

As you gain familiarity, meal planning, recipe adjustments, and restaurant choices will become more intuitive. You'll quickly identify high-risk foods and naturally gravitate toward more filling, balanced meals that keep you satisfied and energized.

Mastering GI and GL is not just about numbers; it's about building a foundation for lasting dietary change. With each meal, you strengthen habits that support your weight loss and overall health.

In the next chapter, we'll dive deeper into how your body processes carbohydrates, the effects of GI and GL on insulin and hunger, and the essential biological links between blood sugar and weight management. For now, keep your GI/GL references handy, and start making every meal with slower, steadier blood sugar in mind. These fundamental skills will serve you well on your journey to better health and sustainable weight loss.

Linking Glycemic Response to Weight Loss Mechanisms

Sustainable energy and effective, long-term weight control start with understanding how your body processes different types of carbohydrates. While Chapter 1 introduced the concepts of glycemic index (GI) and glycemic load (GL), this chapter takes you further, showing exactly how these values influence metabolism, appetite, fat storage, and ultimately your ability to lose or maintain weight.

We'll follow the journey of carbohydrates from the moment they enter your mouth to their impact on your blood sugar, insulin levels, hunger signals, and beyond. By mastering these principles, you'll discover practical ways to curb hunger, avoid cravings, and overcome common diet obstacles especially when reducing calories.

The Metabolic Journey: From Carbohydrate Ingestion to Blood Sugar Fluctuation

Let's begin with a typical breakfast scenario: oatmeal versus white toast with jam. What actually happens inside your body after you eat these foods?

1. ***Ingestion***: You chew and swallow carbohydrate-rich foods such as bread, fruit, starchy vegetables, or sweets.
2. ***Digestion***: Your saliva and digestive enzymes in the small intestine break down complex carbs into simple sugars, mainly glucose.
3. ***Absorption***: Glucose rapidly enters your bloodstream, elevating blood sugar levels.
4. ***Glycemic Response***: Here's where GI and GL come in:
    - High-GI, high-GL foods (like white toast with jam) cause a sharp, rapid spike in blood sugar.
    - Low-GI, low-GL foods (like oatmeal) result in a gradual, moderate rise.

5. ***Insulin Release***: Your pancreas detects the increased glucose and secretes insulin, a hormone that shuttles glucose into cells for energy or stores it as fat if there's excess.
6. ***Blood Sugar Decline and Aftereffects***:
    - ***High-GI foods prompt a big insulin surge***, which can drop blood sugar below your

pre-meal level, leaving you fatigued and hungry again soon after eating.

- ***Low-GI foods lead to a more measured insulin response***, stabilizing blood sugar and supporting longer-lasting fullness and steady energy.

GI/GL, Insulin, and Weight Management: How the Cycle Works

The way your blood sugar changes after eating dictates how much insulin your body produces. This, in turn, impacts your feelings of hunger, your tendency to store fat, and your overall weight outcomes. To see this in action, let's look at a simple table:

Table 2: Sample GI/GL Level Table

Food Type	GI/GL Level	Typical Insulin Response	Likely Weight-Management Effect
White bread, potatoes, sweetened cereals	High	Rapid and pronounced spike	Hunger returns sooner; may encourage overeating and fat storage
Brown rice, pineapple, couscous	Moderate	Moderate, more balanced rise	More satisfying when paired with fiber, protein, or healthy fats
Lentils, beans, non-starchy vegetables	Low	Gradual, steady increase	Promotes fullness, reduces cravings, and supports weight management

The sharper and more dramatic the rise (and subsequent fall) of your blood sugar and insulin, the sooner you'll feel hungry again and the more likely you are to store excess calories as fat. By contrast, low-GI/GL food choices help break this cycle, supporting both weight loss and maintenance.

Hunger, Energy, and Fat Storage: The Real-World Impact of GI and GL

Why do some meals leave you satisfied for hours, while others spark cravings or energy crashes soon after? It comes down to the speed and height of your blood sugar fluctuations:

High-GI/GL foods (such as white bread, sugary cereals, instant potatoes) quickly elevate blood sugar, triggering a strong insulin response. As blood sugar drops, your brain senses an energy shortage, resulting in tiredness, irritability, and a craving for more fast carbs restarting the cycle again.

Low-GI/GL foods (like oats, lentils, and non-starchy vegetables) create a slow, steady rise in blood sugar. Insulin is released gradually, keeping blood sugar stable and hunger suppressed for longer periods.

Low-GI meals also help regulate hunger hormones. For example, they reduce the hunger hormone ghrelin and support higher levels of peptide YY, a hormone that signals fullness. Stable blood sugar means you're less likely to reach for calorie-dense snacks or overeat at the next meal. On the other hand, frequent high-GI meals can overstimulate your insulin response, encouraging the body to store more fat, particularly around the abdominal area, and making weight loss harder even if you're eating fewer calories overall.

Consider these practical examples:

- A breakfast of sugary cereal (high GI) may leave you hungry and low on energy within 90 minutes, increasing the likelihood of impulsive snacking.
- A breakfast of oats with berries and a few nuts (low GI) provides sustained energy and fullness until lunchtime.

This isn't just about physiology, it's psychological as well. Steady blood sugar helps you feel calm and focused, making it easier to stick to your eating plan. High-GI eating, in contrast, can feel like being on a metabolic roller-coaster, undermining willpower and motivation. That's why GI/GL-aware choices lay the foundation for appetite control and steady weight loss.

Choosing Foods for Maximum Satiety During Calorie Reduction

When you're eating fewer calories, managing hunger is critical. Not all carbohydrates, even so-called "healthy carbs" are equally satisfying. Here's how to optimize your food choices for satiety and blood sugar control:

1. ***Low Glycemic Index (<55)***: Center your meals and snacks on low-GI foods like most legumes (lentils, beans), barley, old-fashioned oats, and non-starchy vegetables (broccoli, leafy greens, zucchini).
2. ***Low Glycemic Load***: Aim for servings that keep the glycemic load below about 10–12 per serving—this keeps the total blood sugar impact low, even if the food has some carbohydrate.
3. ***High Fiber Content***: Soluble and insoluble fiber slow digestion, help stabilize blood sugar, and increase fullness. Include plenty of beans, whole fruits (not juice), and high-fiber veggies at every meal.
4. ***Protein and Healthy Fats***: Adding protein (such as eggs, Greek yogurt, fish, lean meats, tofu) and healthy fats (nuts, seeds, olive oil, avocado) further slows the absorption of carbs, blunting blood sugar spikes and prolonging satiety.
5. ***Minimal Processing***: Less processed foods almost always have a lower GI. For instance, choose whole barley over instant barley, or steel-cut oats over instant oatmeal.
6. ***Low Free Sugar***: Foods with added sugars raise GI sharply and are more likely to trigger rapid hunger. Favor naturally sweet foods like fruit instead.
7. ***High Water Content***: Foods with lots of water such as soups, salads, and some fruits and vegetables are more filling with fewer calories and carbs.

A meal designed for appetite control might feature a lentil stew (low GI/GL, high fiber and protein), a leafy green salad dressed with olive oil, and a whole orange or apple for dessert.

Satiety-Supportive, Low-GI Foods—Your Go-To List:

- Oats (regular or steel-cut)
- Lentils, chickpeas, black beans
- Barley, quinoa
- Apples, pears, oranges, berries (whole, not juice)
- Leafy greens, broccoli, zucchini, eggplant
- Plain Greek yogurt, eggs
- Salmon, chicken breast, tofu, edamame

Including these foods in your daily menu makes it easier to reduce calories without suffering from constant hunger or cravings.

Quick-Reference Guide: Symptoms of Poor Blood Sugar Stability

Recognizing signs of unstable blood sugar can help you make timely adjustments to your meals before you experience setbacks. High-GI meals, skipping meals, or eating unbalanced snacks often produce the following symptoms:

Table 3: Quick-Reference Guide

Symptom	Likely Cause	Suggested GI/GL Adjustment
Sudden fatigue or energy crash	Rapid drop in blood sugar after a spike	Replace high-GI carbs with lower-GI options and include protein or fiber
Shakiness or irritability	Strong insulin response leading to low blood sugar	Add protein and fiber to meals; reduce added sugars and refined carbs
Trouble concentrating	Fluctuating blood sugar levels	Pair complex carbohydrates with healthy fats and protein
Persistent hunger or cravings	Repeated blood sugar spikes and dips	Increase fiber and protein; review carbohydrate quality and portion size
Headaches after eating	Blood sugar swings	Choose lower-GI foods and consider smaller, balanced portions
Frequent thirst or urination	Repeated high blood sugar levels	Reduce overall GI/GL load and monitor carbohydrate intake

If you regularly experience these symptoms after meals, it's likely your GI/GL choices need attention. Swapping out high-GI foods like white rice or crackers for beans or barley can correct many of these complaints and help stabilize your energy and appetite.

Practical Example: Solving a Hunger Crash

After a lunch of white bread with turkey, it's common to feel hungry, unfocused, and crave sweets by 3 p.m.—a classic high-GI crash. Here's how to fix it:

- Replace white bread with a low-GI base such as whole-grain rye or, even better, a lentil salad.
- Add high-fiber vegetables and a source of healthy fat, like avocado or olive oil.
- Choose gentle, sustained-release carbs like an apple or carrot sticks for a side.

These simple swaps can help prevent energy swings and promote lasting fullness, making it easier to stick with a calorie-reduced plan.

Tips for Succeeding with GI/GL Strategies

1. ***Plan Meals Ahead***: Choose recipes that feature low-GI staples and plenty of vegetables, legumes, and lean proteins.
2. ***Read Labels Carefully***: Watch for added sugars even in foods marketed as healthy.
3. ***Balance Plates***: Always include a mix of protein, healthy fat, and fiber-rich carbs to slow digestion and buffer any glycemic impact.
4. ***Mind Portions***: Even healthy carbs can spike your blood sugar if you eat too much at once. Pay attention to serving sizes, especially for rice, bread, pasta, and fruit.
5. ***Stay Consistent***: Making low-GI/GL choices part of your daily routine leads to more stable energy and less temptation to overeat.

6. ***Listen to Your Body***: Use the symptom matrix to spot patterns. If you feel unwell after certain meals, experiment with lowering the GI/GL and adjusting your combinations.

Effective weight regulation depends not just on what and how much you eat, but also on how quickly those foods are digested and metabolized. Glycemic index and load provide a practical framework for connecting your food choices with real metabolic outcomes: low-GI/GL foods support satiety, steady energy, and lower fat storage, while high-GI foods trigger insulin surges, blood sugar drops, and cravings that can derail your weight loss efforts even if you're eating less overall.

Use the GI/GL grid and symptom matrix as everyday tools to build meals that keep you satisfied and energized. Treat every meal as fuel for stable metabolism, and don't be afraid to adjust your menu if you notice hunger or energy problems cropping up.

In the next chapter, you'll learn how to assemble low-GI meals, select ingredients that tame appetite, and create a daily menu that helps you power through energy dips and resist temptations. Keep your GI/GL guidelines and satiety strategies close at hand because with the right approach, satisfying and effective calorie control is possible at every meal.

Stepwise Method for Low-GI Meal Construction

Sustaining a low-GI diet involves more than identifying foods that raise blood sugar. Weight control and stable energy depend on building balanced meals with every eating occasion. This chapter presents a step-by-step system to assemble meals that maximize low-glycemic impact, simplify ingredient choices, reduce pitfalls, and keep portions reasonable for calorie management. The following framework supports both daily cooking and batching for the week.

Low-GI Plate Assembly Framework

Use a structured approach to plate building so every meal features nutrient-rich, low-GI foods from key food groups, slowing glucose absorption and extending fullness. This framework guides any meal:

- Begin with non-starchy vegetables or leafy greens as the plate's core.
- Add a moderate amount of low-GI, high-fiber carbs, whole grains (barley, quinoa), lentils, or beans.

- Include lean protein sources such as fish, chicken, tofu, eggs, or Greek yogurt.
- Add measured healthy fats: olive oil, avocado, seeds, or nuts.
- Use fruit as a side or dessert; stick to whole, low-GI fruits, not juice or dried forms.
- Minimize salt, added sugar, and sauces; season with herbs and spices.

This balanced model reduces glycemic load: non-starchy vegetables provide ample volume with little blood sugar impact, and pairing carbs with protein and fat further blunts post-meal spikes.

A sample low-GI breakfast could be a spinach and tomato omelet (vegetables/protein), a small bowl of steel-cut oats (low-GI carb), and a sprinkle of nuts (healthy fat). For lunch, leafy greens with chickpeas, roasted eggplant, and tahini-lemon dressing hit all targets. A low-GI dinner might feature grilled salmon, quinoa, sautéed broccoli, and a few orange slices.

Ingredient Selection Checklist with GI/GL Targets

Careful food selection grounds effective low-GI meals. Here's a checklist and GI/GL targets for each meal element:

Carbohydrate Source:

- Choose main starch sources with GI ≤55: barley, lentils, black beans, old-fashioned oats, or whole cooked sweet potatoes with skin.
- Aim for a glycemic load (GL) per carb portion ≤10 to ensure a mild overall glycemic effect.
- Restrict moderate GI foods (GI 56–69) to occasional, half-size servings, and pair with extra fiber/protein.

Protein and Fat:

- Add minimally processed lean protein eggs, fish, skinless poultry, tofu, and legumes. These lower GI's impact and boost satiety.
- Favor unsaturated fats avocado, olive oil, nuts, and seeds that slow digestion and glucose uptake.

Vegetables and Fruits:

- Choose non-starchy vegetables (often GI <30) for at least a third to half of your plate.
- For fruit, pick low-GI types like apples, pears, oranges, and berries. Serve whole to retain fiber.

Breads and Grains:

- If eating bread, choose dense, minimally processed, whole-grain, or sprouted kinds with visible grains or seeds; rye or pumpernickel and stone-ground whole wheat have lower GI.

- Limit to one slice or at most a quarter of your plate.

Miscellaneous:

- Avoid foods with sugars (sucrose, glucose syrup, etc.) among the first three ingredients.
- Read labels to prefer high-fiber (>3g/serving) and low-added-sugar items.

Survey each meal with this list. If more than one ingredient is high-GI, replace one with a low-GI alternative. Over time, this habit will make balanced, low-GI eating effortless and routine.

Rule-Setting for Hidden Sugars and High-GI Starches in Mixed Dishes

Mixed dishes, stir-fries, casseroles, grain bowls often hide high-GI starches or added sugars. Maintain control using these rules:

- ***Starches***: Include only ONE carbohydrate component per mixed dish with a GI less than 55 (e.g., brown lentils, quinoa, barley). Do not combine multiple high-GI grains or roots like white rice and potatoes.
- ***Portion Limits***: Cap rice, pasta, or bread at half-cup cooked per person, and buffer with beans or vegetables.
- ***Hidden Sugars***: Check sauces/dressings/marinades for sugar; opt for from-scratch versions with little or no

added sugar, or store-bought with ≤2g sugar/tablespoon, using minimally.

- ***Canned or Prepared Goods***: Select "no added sugar" or "unsweetened" versions. Rinse canned items to remove syrups or starchy brine.
- ***Fast Carbs***: Avoid high-GI "convenience" carbs like instant couscous, processed cereals, and mashed potatoes, swapping in slow-digesting grains or legumes.

For example, in chili, use just enough canned tomatoes for flavor but emphasize black beans and vegetables over corn or thickeners. In pasta, use moderate noodles, double the vegetables, and add protein (chicken or lentils).

Batch-Cooking Efficiency for Low-GI Eating

Batch-cooking makes it much easier to sustain low-GI eating during busy weeks. Follow this efficient prep sequence:

1. ***Prep Base Components***: Batch-cook low-GI staples: dry beans/lentils, brown or wild rice, roasted non-starchy vegetables, and lean proteins (grilled chicken, eggs).
2. ***Cooking Sequence***: Start grains or beans first (longest cooking). While they cook, roast/steam vegetables. Simultaneously, prep protein, bake salmon, poach eggs, or grill tofu.
3. ***Organize for Flexibility***:

- Store components separately (grains, beans, veggies, proteins) for mix-and-match variety.
- Pre-make simple, low-sugar dressings.
- Portion low-GI fruit for snacks.

4. ***Assembly***:
   - For each meal, combine at least one protein, one low-GI carb, and two or more non-starchy vegetables, topped with healthy fat.
   - Rotate seasonings and sides to keep meals interesting.

5. ***Time-Saving Tips:***
   - Freeze portions of cooked beans or grains to save time and expand options.
   - Use pre-washed greens or frozen, unseasoned vegetables for quicker assembly.

Prepping these basics, you're equipped to avoid last-minute, high-GI decisions, always having the essentials ready for balanced meals.

Portion Guide for Calorie and GI Control

Managing glycemic index ensures stable energy, but calorie control is key for weight loss. Use this rule set to keep both in check:

1. **Visual Plate Guide:**
   - Fill half your plate with non-starchy vegetables.

- Limit low-GI grains/starchy carbs to one quarter (size of a cupped hand).
- Allocate one quarter to protein (palm-sized).
- Add 1–2 tablespoons of healthy fat (e.g., olive oil) per meal.

2. **Tailor to Activity:**
    - Increase carbs slightly on active days, but stick to low-GI sources.
    - For less activity or faster weight loss, reduce carbs and increase vegetables and protein.

3. **Monitor Glycemic Load:**

    Large portions increase GL. Keep total meal GL under 20, snacks under 10.

4. **Mindful Eating:**
    - Start with modest portions; wait 10–15 minutes before seconds, since low-GI meals can take time to curb hunger.
    - Drink water and eat with minimal distractions.

5. **Smart Snacks:**

    Pair low-GI carbs with protein and fat: e.g., Greek yogurt with berries, bean dip with carrots, or an apple with nut butter.

6. **Track and Tweak:**

   Log food, portions, and hunger/satiety. Adjust ratios if consistently too full or hungry.

If you feel sluggish mid-afternoon, revisit lunch: was the carb portion correct and low-GI, protein sufficient? Adjust for future meals as needed.

Practical Example: Low-GI Lunch

1. Fill half a plate with salad greens, cherry tomatoes, cucumber, and roasted peppers.
2. Add 1/2 cup cooked lentils (low-GI carb).
3. Top with grilled chicken (protein) and a tablespoon of walnuts (healthy fat).
4. Side of orange wedges (low-GI fruit).
5. Dress with olive oil, lemon, pepper, herbs to avoid sugary dressings.
6. Log to ensure low-GI carbs, GL under 20, ample veggies, and right portion sizes.

If more calories are needed (e.g., after exercise), slightly increase lentils or chicken rather than adding white bread.

Troubleshooting and Adjusting

If meals leave you hungry, craving, or tired, reassess:

- Was the main carb low-GI?
- Were at least half the plate vegetables?
- Was protein sufficient (palm size)?

- Keep fats to no more than 2 tablespoons?
- Avoided high-GI starches, juice, and sugary extras?

Targeted tweaks to ingredients, portions, or meal structure resolve most satiety and calorie concerns.

Constructing low-GI, weight-loss-supporting meals becomes simple with this systematic approach: follow plate assembly guidelines, select ingredients with care, control hidden sugars, use batch prep, and adjust portions to match your needs. By doing so, you sustain progress, avoid typical setbacks, and achieve lasting success with a low-GI lifestyle.

High-GI Food Swaps for Everyday Eating

Transitioning to a low-glycemic-index (GI) diet is not about adhering to strict lists of "good" and "bad" foods. Instead, it is about developing practical and manageable strategies that fit seamlessly into everyday life. This is especially relevant when dealing with common high-GI staples, navigating busy schedules, and eating out at restaurants or social gatherings.

By focusing on intentional swaps rather than outright eliminations, you can effectively manage blood sugar and weight while still enjoying your meals. This chapter provides a comprehensive framework to make low-GI living practical through simple swaps, smarter shopping, thoughtful cooking methods, and adaptable choices in any setting.

Understanding the Importance of Food Swaps

Many common meal staples such as white bread, instant rice, most cereals, and potatoes can cause rapid spikes and crashes in blood sugar, affecting energy levels and appetite. Fortunately, nearly every high-GI food has an accessible and tasty low-GI substitute. Reconfiguring your meals with these alternatives helps support steadier blood sugar and longer-lasting satiety.

The Swap Guide: Everyday High-GI Staples and Their Low-GI Alternatives

Below is a practical swap matrix to help you identify opportunities to substitute high-GI foods with better options throughout the day. Use it as a reference to make gradual, sustainable changes.

Breakfast:

- ***High-GI***: Cornflakes, puffed rice cereal, instant oatmeal, white toast
- ***Swap for***: Steel-cut or old-fashioned oats, natural muesli, Greek yogurt topped with berries, dense whole-grain toast
- ***High-GI***: Fruit juice and sweetened smoothies
- ***Swap for***: Whole fruit such as apples, pears, or berries, and unsweetened yogurt with a handful of nuts and seeds

Lunch:

- ***High-GI***: White bread, instant noodles, fries, pretzels
- ***Swap for***: Whole grain or rye bread, quinoa, barley, lentil salad, baked sweet potato, air-popped popcorn without added sugar
- ***High-GI***: Flavored or fruit-on-the-bottom yogurt

- ***Swap for***: Plain Greek yogurt flavored with cinnamon and fresh fruit

Dinner:

- ***High-GI***: White rice, instant mashed potatoes, white pasta
- ***Swap for***: Brown or wild rice, farro, bulgur, lentils, chickpeas, roasted root vegetables, spiralized zucchini noodles
- ***High-GI***: Regular-crust pizza
- ***Swap for***: Homemade pizza using whole grain or legume-based crusts topped with vegetables and lean proteins

Snacks:

- ***High-GI***: Potato chips, rice cakes, sports bars
- ***Swap for***: Hummus with vegetable sticks, unsalted nuts, roasted chickpeas, apple slices with almond butter, oat or nut flour-based mini muffins

Desserts:

- ***High-GI***: Store-bought cakes, cookies, donuts
- ***Swap for***: Low-sugar oatmeal-raisin cookies, baked apples with cinnamon, chia pudding with berries

This flexible matrix allows you to spot swap opportunities across all meals, replacing fast-digesting starches and sugars with slower-digesting options that help sustain energy. Over time, these choices become routine, helping to anchor stable blood glucose and simplify weight management.

Ingredient Shopping Template: Upgrading Your Pantry for Success

A low-GI lifestyle starts at the grocery store. Stocking the right supplies makes healthy swaps easier and more automatic. Use the following shopping template as a guide for your next trip:

Whole Grains and Pulses:

- Purchase steel-cut or old-fashioned oats instead of instant varieties
- Select bulgur, barley, farro, brown, black, or red rice in place of white or instant rice
- Stock up on canned or dried lentils, chickpeas, and black beans (remember to rinse canned beans before use)
- Choose sprouted, rye, or pumpernickel bread, looking for visible grains and minimal sugar

Non-Starchy Vegetables:

Fill your cart with leafy greens, broccoli, cauliflower, bell peppers, zucchini, eggplant, tomatoes, and cucumber

Fruits:

Prioritize apples, oranges, pears, berries, peaches, and plums over higher-GI options such as bananas or watermelon

Protein Sources:

Include eggs, plain Greek yogurt, tofu, tempeh, skinless poultry or fish, and unsalted nuts and seeds

Healthy Fats and Condiments:

Select extra-virgin olive oil, avocados, vinegar, mustard, hummus, and salsa

Baking and Snacks:

- Use nut flours such as almond or coconut instead of refined flours for baking
- Purchase popcorn kernels (not pre-flavored), dried chickpeas, or edamame for roasting at home

Stocking these basics steers your eating toward lower-GI options throughout the week. Organizing your shopping list by these groups and focusing your shopping around the store's perimeter can help reduce the temptation to pick up processed, high-GI snacks.

Cooking Modification Chart: Lowering GI Through Preparation Methods

How you prepare and cook your food can impact its glycemic index as much as the ingredients you choose. Adapting your cooking methods can help lower the glycemic impact of meals, even when using the same basic ingredients. Consider the following suggestions:

Starches, Rice, and Pasta:

- Cook pasta and barley until just tender (al dente) to keep their GI lower
- Cool and reheat rice or potatoes to increase resistant starch, which helps lower their GI
- Opt for whole, intact grains instead of those that are ground or flaked

Vegetables:

- Roast or bake vegetables with their skins on to retain fiber and reduce the rise in GI
- Roasting or grilling helps preserve the structure of vegetables, resulting in a gentler impact on blood sugar than boiling

Legumes:

- Rinse canned beans to lower added starch and sodium
- Slow-cook beans to boost resistant starch; avoid overcooking or pureeing them

Breads and Muffins:

Use batters made with whole grains, and add in nuts, seeds, or grated vegetables to increase fiber and lower GI

Fruit:

Serve whole fruit with the skin rather than as juices, sauces, or sweetened dried versions

Snacks and Sweets:

Pair carbohydrates with protein or fat, such as apple slices with nut butter, crackers with cheese, or yogurt with seeds, to blunt post-meal sugar spikes

Small changes in cooking methods can yield lasting benefits for metabolic health and weight control.

Flavor-Matching and Texture-Based Substitutions: Satisfaction Without Sacrifice

A common concern is that low-GI foods will taste bland or lack the comforting textures of familiar favorites. You can address these cravings by choosing swaps that match the desired texture and flavor profile:

1. For a crispy or crunchy experience, trade chips for roasted chickpeas, mixed nuts, air-popped popcorn, or seed-based crackers.
2. To satisfy creamy or rich cravings, use plain Greek yogurt with berries, cinnamon, or unsweetened

coconut as an alternative to sweetened yogurts and desserts.

3. For sweet cravings, try overnight oats with spices, apples, and nuts, or bake fruit with cinnamon and nuts for a naturally sweet dessert.
4. When you want comfort starches, build stews or chilis around lentils or beans. Mash cauliflower or white beans as a lower-GI alternative to mashed potatoes, or use whole grain or lentil pasta for "mac and cheese" dishes.
5. To address salty or savory cravings, enjoy olives, cheese, pickled vegetables, or hummus with sliced raw vegetables.
6. For texture tweaks, add pumpkin seeds or roasted edamame for crunch, or use avocado or blended cottage cheese for creaminess.

Focusing on what you are adding in terms of flavor and enjoyment, not just what you are removing, you will find that a lower-GI approach can be enjoyable as well as sustainable.

"Swap It or Skip It" Guide: Making Smart Choices When Eating Out

Eating out or grabbing takeout often presents high-GI temptations. The following quick guide can help you make informed swaps and minimize the glycemic impact:

Bread and Appetizers:

- Swap: Ask for whole-grain or rye bread and request olive oil for dipping
- Skip: White rolls, crackers, or breadsticks

Salads and Bowls:

- Swap: Choose salads with beans, nuts, plenty of vegetables, and oil-based dressings
- Skip: Salads with crispy noodles, sweetened dried fruit, croutons, or sugary dressings

Main Courses:

- Swap: Select grilled or roasted proteins served with lots of vegetables; look for grain or pulse bowls featuring quinoa, lentils, or barley
- Skip: Deep-fried or battered proteins, and main dishes based on refined pasta or white rice

Side Dishes:

- Swap: Order beans, lentil soup, grilled vegetables, side salads, or baked sweet potatoes with the skin on
- Skip: Fries, mashed potatoes, or white and sticky rice

Snacks and Convenience Foods:

- Swap: Choose trail mix made from nuts, seeds, and unsweetened dried fruit, plain yogurt, hard-boiled eggs, or hummus with veggie sticks

- Skip: Rice-based granola bars, fried chips, sweet pastries, or packaged muffins

Quick Restaurant Tips:

- If bread can be easily squashed between two fingers, it is likely high-GI; denser, seedier breads are generally better choices
- Ask for a serving of protein along with at least two servings of vegetables. If not included, request extra sides to round out your meal

Reading Packaged Snack Labels:

- Choose products with more than 3 grams of fiber per serving and less than 2 grams of added sugar per serving for the best options
- Look for whole foods as the first ingredients, such as "whole oats" or "chickpeas."

Whenever possible, modify menu orders by going "no bun," swapping a salad for fries, or doubling up on vegetables. These strategies help you control your glycemic impact in social or fast-food settings with minimal extra effort.

Mealtime offers countless opportunities for strategic swaps that can positively influence your health. Maintain a mental or written swap chart and shopping template, prepare low-GI staples in batches, modify your cooking techniques, and choose flavor-matched alternatives to make healthier choices easier. The "Swap It or Skip It" guide will support your weight and energy goals, wherever you choose to eat.

Try dedicating a week to conscious swaps, tracking which alternatives are most satisfying for you. With time, these choices will become second nature, supporting long-term health, expanding your enjoyment of food, and sustaining your progress. The next chapter will provide a ready-to-use 7-day meal plan to put these strategies into daily action, complete with recipes and practical tips for busy schedules.

7-Day Low-GI Weight Loss Meal Plan

A week-long low-glycemic-index (GI) meal plan helps turn healthy choices into daily habits rather than occasional efforts. By focusing on structured meals, varied ingredients, time-saving batch prep, and balanced nutrients, you support weight loss while enjoying satisfying food each day. This chapter provides a practical guide to translate low-GI principles into actionable, repeatable routines.

Daily Menu Table: Breakfast, Lunch, Dinner, Snack Structure

An effective low-GI meal plan should provide steady energy and manage hunger by combining slow-digesting carbohydrates with lean proteins, healthy fats, and fiber-rich vegetables. Consistent meal and snack times also reduce the risk of impulsive, high-GI eating.

Day 1

- ***Breakfast***: Steel-cut oats with diced apple, walnuts, and cinnamon.

- ***Morning Snack***: Plain Greek yogurt with blueberries and chia seeds.
- ***Lunch***: Lentil and mixed vegetable salad (arugula, cherry tomatoes, cucumber) with lemon-olive oil dressing and a side of almonds.
- ***Afternoon Snack***: Sliced red bell pepper with hummus.
- ***Dinner***: Grilled salmon, roasted Brussels sprouts, farro, and mixed greens with vinaigrette.

Days 2–7 repeat this structure:

- ***Breakfast***: Whole-grain or protein-rich base muesli, eggs with spinach, or overnight oats with pear and pumpkin seeds.
- ***Snacks***: Unsweetened yogurt, fruit (berries, orange, plum), nuts, or veggie sticks with hummus or guacamole.
- ***Lunch***: Pulses, whole grains (quinoa, barley, brown rice), leafy greens, non-starchy vegetables, and a protein (beans, eggs, tuna, tofu).
- ***Dinner***: Rotated proteins (chicken, fish, lentils, or tempeh) with vegetables, whole grains, or legumes.

Predictable meal rhythms promote consistency and better metabolic outcomes.

GI/GL Meal Calculator Template

Calculating both glycemic index (GI) and glycemic load (GL) for each meal promotes blood sugar stability and aligns carbohydrate intake with weight loss goals.

Steps to apply this approach:

Assign GI values to each ingredient using a trusted database. For example:

- Steel-cut oats (GI 52), apple (GI 36), walnuts (GI ~15), yogurt (GI 47), chickpeas (GI 28), brown rice (GI 50).
- Calculate GL: Multiply carb grams per serving by GI, then divide by 100 (Carbs × GI ÷ 100 = GL).
- Sum the GLs for all foods in a meal.
- Keep total meal GL in the "low" (10 or below) to "moderate" (11–19) range; most meals should stay under GL 20. Snacks ideally have a GL of 5–10 or less.

Breakfast example:

- 1/2 cup steel-cut oats (24g carbs × 52 GI ÷ 100 = 12.5 GL)
- 1/2 apple (10g carbs × 36 GI ÷ 100 = 3.6 GL)
- 1 Tbsp walnuts (1g carb × 15 GI ÷ 100 = 0.15 GL)
- Total meal GL ≈ 16.25 (moderate)

Use a simple worksheet to enter ingredients and visualize your glycemic impact. Adjust portions, swap foods, or tweak combinations to keep meals within GL targets.

Rotating Ingredient Planner for GI-Friendly Variety

Dietary variety prevents monotony and increases nutrient diversity. A rotating ingredient planner keeps meals interesting without increasing GI.

Structure your weekly rotation as follows:

Grains and Pseudo-Grains (Low to Moderate GI):

- Oats (steel-cut, rolled)
- barley
- bulgur
- quinoa brown/black/red rice
- farro

Legumes and Pulses:

- Lentils
- black beans
- chickpeas
- kidney beans

Vegetables:

- Leafy greens (spinach, kale, arugula),
- cruciferous (broccoli, cauliflower, Brussels sprouts),

- peppers,
- zucchini,
- eggplant,
- tomatoes
- carrots

Fruits (Low-GI Picks):

- Apples,
- pears
- oranges
- plums
- berries
- peaches
- grapefruit

Proteins:

- Eggs
- fish (salmon, sardines, cod)
- poultry
- tofu
- tempeh
- unsalted nuts/seeds

Healthy Fats:

- Extra-virgin olive oil
- avocado
- nut butters

- flax/chia seeds

Select two to three items from each group per week and change combinations daily to maximize variety and maintain a low-GI profile. This system also simplifies shopping and streamlines meal prep, supporting optimal nutrition.

Advance Batch-Prep Timeline for Success

Proper preparation is key to following any meal plan. Batch-prepping once or twice weekly eliminates last-minute reliance on high-GI options and ensures healthy, ready-to-eat meals.

Weekly batch-prep example:

Weekend (Before Start):

- Prepare large batches of whole grains (quinoa, brown rice, barley) for breakfasts and sides.
- Cook lentils or chickpeas for lunches/dinners.
- Roast a tray of mixed vegetables (peppers, cauliflower, zucchini, carrots).
- Wash and chop leafy greens (spinach, kale, arugula).
- Boil or bake eggs for breakfasts/snacks.
- Portion Greek yogurt and berries into containers for snacks.

Mid-Week (Mini Batch-Prep):

- Replenish roasted veggies and cooked grains.

- Prepare extra hummus or nut butter spreads.
- Wash fruit and restock snack containers.

Ongoing:

- Each evening, assemble salad jars or bento boxes for the next day using pre-made components.
- Refresh vinaigrettes every few days.

Storage tips:

- Keep cooked grains and beans in airtight containers for up to four days; freeze extras.
- Stock quick proteins (canned tuna, rotisserie chicken, tofu) to mix with prepped items.

Batch-prepping creates versatile meal components, not identical meals, making it easy to assemble creative, low-GI dishes ensuring that healthy choices are always the easiest option.

Weekly Nutrient Balance Scorecard: Fiber, Protein, and Micronutrient Benchmarks

Weight loss and good health depend on balancing glycemic control with adequate fiber, protein, and essential micronutrients.

Use this daily checklist to gauge nutritional balance:

1. **Fiber:**
    - Target 25–35 grams per day from vegetables, fruits, whole grains, legumes, and seeds.
    - Track fiber sources at each meal; emphasize vegetables or legumes at lunch/dinner, fruit/whole grains at breakfast/snacks.

    Example: Salad with lentils, peppers, greens and an apple as a snack can provide 12–15 grams at one meal.

2. **Protein:**
    - Target 15–25 grams per meal, 5–10 grams per snack, depending on needs and activity.
    - Include a protein (beans, fish, eggs, Greek yogurt, tofu, nuts) in every meal/snack.
3. **Micronutrients:**
    - Prioritize magnesium, potassium, zinc, B vitamins, and antioxidants from varied plant foods, legumes, nuts, and whole grains.
    - Each day, include three or more colors of produce, rotating leafy greens, cruciferous veggies, and citrus or berries.

    Example: Lunch mixed greens, red tomatoes, yellow peppers; Dinner—roasted purple carrots, orange salmon.

Table 4: Sample Scorecard (fill out at day's end):

Habit Check	Yes	No
Ate 5+ servings of non-starchy vegetables	☐	☐
Had 2–3 servings of low-GI fruit	☐	☐
Included protein at every meal	☐	☐
Ate at least 2 servings of legumes/pulses	☐	☐
Choose snacks with at least 5 g fiber	☐	☐
Included healthy fats (nuts, seeds, olive oil, etc.)	☐	☐
Ate three or more different-colored fruits/vegetables	☐	☐
Choose whole, low-GI grains or major carbs	☐	☐
Ate at least one batch-prepped or planned meal	☐	☐

Consistently checking these boxes ensures balanced nutrition all week. This integrated focus supports weight loss, improves energy, reduces cravings, and supports long-term health.

Practical Example: Daily Implementation

- On Monday, start with overnight oats (rolled oats, chia, diced pear, almond milk) and a hard-boiled egg.
- For a morning snack, have Greek yogurt and strawberries. Lunch is a bento with barley, roasted broccoli, lentil salad, greens, and hummus.
- Afternoon snack: bell pepper strips with chickpea dip.
- Dinner: roasted chicken, sweet potatoes (with skin), and spinach-walnut salad—mostly batch-prepped or quickly assembled.

Track each meal's GI/GL using your calculator and check fiber/protein/produce intake on your scorecard. For variety, switch up lunch proteins or greens, or snack on oranges instead of berries. Batch-cooked proteins and grains keep meal assembly quick and flexible.

Through the week, repeat structure while adjusting ingredients—creating an easy, automatic rhythm for low-GI eating.

While planning and prep are vital, so is flexibility. Make substitutions if ingredients run low or your tastes change. Repeat favorite meals when pressed for time, or use leftovers to minimize waste.

This 7-day template blends GI/GL management, ingredient rotation, batch-prep, and nutrient tracking for both weight loss and lasting healthier eating. As these methods become routine, low-GI living turns into an enjoyable, sustainable part of daily life.

Core Pantry and Shopping System for Low-GI Success

A well-organized pantry forms the foundation of a successful low-GI lifestyle. Transforming your kitchen into a space that supports steady energy and satiety begins with understanding what to buy, how to interpret labels, and how to set up efficient storage. The following outlines the key elements for effective low-GI shopping and pantry management, ensuring that every meal and snack contributes to weight loss and improved well-being.

Core Grocery List by GI/GL Ranking and Shelf Life

A practical low-GI pantry centers on "low" GI foods (GI under 55) and ideally those with low glycemic load (GL). Organizing ingredients by shelf life aids in simplifying shopping and reducing food waste.

Long shelf life (1 month to 1 year or more):

- ***Whole grains***: Steel-cut oats, barley, quinoa, brown/wild rice, farro, bulgur wheat (low-moderate GI, fiber-rich).
- ***Dried legumes***: Lentils, black beans, chickpeas, kidney beans, split peas (low GI, high protein and fiber).
- ***Shelf-stable nuts/seeds***: Walnuts, almonds, chia, flaxseeds, pumpkin seeds (very low GI when unsweetened/unsalted).
- ***Nut butters***: Natural almond and peanut butter without added sugar.
- ***Canned foods***: Beans (rinsed), wild salmon, sardines in water, tuna in brine (protein, low GI).
- ***Whole grain pasta***: Varieties made from lentils, chickpeas, or 100% whole wheat.

Medium shelf life (up to 3 weeks):

- ***Root vegetables***: Sweet potatoes, carrots, beets (lower GI when roasted/baked whole).
- ***Winter squash***: Butternut, acorn, spaghetti (moderate GI, high fiber).
- Apples, pears, oranges, grapefruit (all low GI; store in a cool place).
- Eggs and firm tofu (protein sources, store for weeks if refrigerated).

Short shelf life (up to 1 week):

- ***Leafy greens***: Spinach, kale, romaine, arugula.
- ***Cruciferous vegetables*** include options such as broccoli, cauliflower, and Brussels sprouts.
- ***Summer berries***: Strawberries, blackberries, blueberries, raspberries (low GI, fiber, antioxidants).
- Tomatoes, zucchini, bell peppers, eggplant.

Restock by replacing depleted items, especially in the long and medium shelf-life categories. This makes weekly produce trips easier and ensures meals are anchored in low-GI grains, legumes, and plant foods with a rotating selection of fresh fruits and vegetables for micronutrient variety.

Label Decoding for GI/GL in Packaged Foods

Packaged foods rarely display GI, but a systematic approach enables wise choices for low-GI eating.

A step-by-step decision tree for packaged foods:

1. **Read the Ingredients List:**
    - Favor products where the first three ingredients are whole foods: whole grains, legumes, or nuts.
    - Avoid sugar, glucose, maltodextrin, or high-fructose corn syrup high on the list.

2. **Review the Nutrition Facts:**
    - Compare serving size to total carbs look for higher fiber, lower sugar.

- For grains/crackers/bread, choose options with at least 3g fiber per serving.
- Prefer 0g added sugar and avoid items above 2–3g per serving.

3. **Check for "whole" keywords and certifications:**

   "100% whole grain," "no added sugar," "sprouted grain," "unsweetened" on packaging indicate better choices.

4. **Research GI values:**
   - Leading diabetes and health organizations often publish GI rankings for popular brands online.
   - Favor minimally processed options:
   - Less processing usually equals lower GI; e.g., steel-cut oats (GI 52) versus instant oats (GI 79).

Practicing these steps allows you to quickly assess GI/GL impact and avoid hidden sugars or high-GI starches, making adherence to your plan easier at home and when out.

Bulk Purchasing Guidelines for Low-GI Staples

Buying in bulk lowers costs and ensures healthy ingredients are always available. Focus on foods that stay nutritious over time and are easy to prepare.

Best bulk picks:

- ***Dried legumes***: Lentils, black beans, chickpeas last long, offer high nutrition, and cook in batches. Store in airtight jars.
- ***Whole grains***: Steel-cut oats, brown rice, barley, quinoa; keep in cool, dry places. Freezing unopened bags extends life and deters pests.
- ***Nuts and seeds***: Unsalted, unsweetened types in large containers. Portion out weekly and freeze extras (vital for fatty seeds like flax and chia).
- ***Canned products***: Beans and wild fish—buy multi-packs if space allows.
- ***Frozen low-GI fruit/veg***: Berries, spinach, broccoli, riced cauliflower are handy for smoothies or cooking, and nutrition is nearly equal to fresh.
- ***Batch-prep containers***: Invest in glass or BPA-free containers for storing cooked grains, legumes, and prepped vegetables.

Plan bulk buys by how quickly you use items and available pantry space. Label with purchase dates and rotate stock, using older items first. This approach saves money and reduces fallback to high-GI convenience foods when the fridge is sparse.

Storage and Preparation for High-Satiety, Low-GI Snacks

Having ready, protein- and fiber-rich snacks is essential for a low-GI lifestyle. A simple storage and prep routine makes healthy snacks as convenient as pre-packaged alternatives.

- ***Snack-packing steps***: Set aside fridge and pantry space for low-GI snacks.
- ***Fridge***: Portions of Greek yogurt, cut vegetables, hummus or bean dip cups, hard-boiled eggs, cottage cheese, or tempeh stored in individual containers.
- ***Pantry***: Single-serve packs of unsalted nuts, chia pudding, roasted chickpeas, high-fiber crackers.

Weekly prep:

- Spend 10–15 minutes washing/slicing fruit and veg and packing into portions after shopping.
- Batch-make dips like hummus, white bean or lentil spreads, and guacamole to last 3–5 days.
- Prep overnight oats or chia pudding in jars ahead for the week.
- Assemble snack "kits":
- Pair crackers with nut butter, apple with almonds, or carrots with hummus to combine protein and fiber for satiety.

Use visual cues:

Place healthy snacks at the front of shelves; less desirable items go out of sight.

With this system, you minimize the appeal of processed, high-GI snacks and shape habits toward choices that sustain you.

Budget-Friendly Tips for Affordable Low-GI Grocery Shopping

Eating a low-GI diet doesn't have to break the bank if you plan ahead. Here are some strategies to help you shop smart and save money:

1. **Plan Before You Shop:**
   - Make a weekly meal plan and shopping list, focusing on ingredients that can be used in multiple recipes.
   - Use up pantry staples purchased in bulk before buying more.
2. **Shop Strategically:**
   - Start with dry goods like grains, beans, and nuts, then add produce and proteins that are on sale.
   - Avoid the snack aisles preparing your own snacks is cheaper and healthier.

3. **Prioritize Protein and Fiber:**
    - Choose legumes as an affordable source of low-GI protein and fiber.
    - Buy large packs of eggs or Greek yogurt for easy, low-GI meals and snacks.

4. **Choose Frozen Produce:**

    Frozen fruits and vegetables are often less expensive than fresh and help reduce food waste.

5. **Bulk Buy Staples, Limit Perishable Treats:**

    Buy staple foods in bulk, but purchase perishables in smaller amounts to avoid overspending and spoilage.

6. **Look for Sales and Use Loyalty Programs:**

    Stock up on your core low-GI staples during sales, and join store loyalty programs for extra savings.

7. **Buy Discounted or "Imperfect" Produce:**

    Take advantage of reduced-price fruits and vegetables that are just as nutritious as their perfect counterparts.

Sample budget week: Base meals on bulk lentils, steel-cut oats, and brown rice. Supplement with seasonal apples, spinach, and eggs. Frozen mixed berries and broccoli work for smoothies and dinners; bulk nuts serve as snacks; canned wild salmon or sardines add extra protein variety.

With this approach, the menu remains nutrient-dense, varied, and cost-effective, generally less expensive than a diet based on convenience foods. Consistently checking inventory, planning for overlap in meals, and shopping for sales make low-GI eating both sustainable and affordable.

Mastering your pantry and shopping systems is essential for ongoing low-GI success. By stocking your kitchen with well-chosen, low-GI staples organized for easy access, ready for quick meals and snacks, and shopped for with an eye on both GI and cost you ensure every food choice propels you toward greater energy and your health goals. Using ingredient lists to interpret labels, bulk purchasing essentials, prepping grab-and-go options, and sticking to a mindful budget all work together to make low-GI eating automatic.

As these systems become habits, your daily food decisions grow easier and align with your intentions turning healthy eating from effort into second nature.

Low-GI Weight Loss Recipes

Low-glycemic index (low-GI) recipes promote sustained energy, minimize hunger swings, and support steady weight loss. This chapter presents carefully selected recipes designed to keep blood sugar stable while delivering flavor and satisfaction. Each recipe includes a concise culinary index card listing ingredients, GI and GL values, prep time, and servings, plus clear instructions for preparation, customization, and troubleshooting to maintain their low-GI status.

Culinary Index Cards: Quick-Glance Nutrition

- Each recipe is paired with an index card containing:
- Ingredient list featuring low- or moderate-GI foods
- Estimated GI for main carbohydrates
- Glycemic Load (GL) per serving
- Prep time (active and total)
- Default servings

Sample index card:

- ***Ingredients***: Green lentils, carrots, celery, tomatoes, spinach, onions, garlic, olive oil, cumin, black pepper
- ***Main Carb GI***: Lentils ~32
- ***GL/serving***: ~9
- ***Prep***: 10 min prep, 40 min simmer
- ***Servings***: 4

These index cards help you plan meals and quickly gauge how each recipe aligns with your target eating plan using GI and GL estimates.

Low-GI Weight Loss Recipe

Steel-Cut Oat & Berry Breakfast Bowl

Ingredients:

- 1 cup steel-cut oats
- 1/2 cup blueberries (fresh or frozen)
- 1 tablespoon chia seeds
- 1/2 cup Greek yogurt
- 1/2 teaspoon cinnamon

Instructions:

1. Bring 3 cups of water to a boil in a saucepan. Add steel-cut oats and reduce heat to low. Simmer for 20–25 minutes, stirring occasionally, until oats are tender.
2. Divide the cooked oats between two bowls.
3. Top each bowl with blueberries, chia seeds, Greek yogurt, and a sprinkle of cinnamon.
4. Serve warm.

Savory Veggie Omelet

Ingredients:

- 2 eggs
- 1/2 cup fresh spinach, chopped
- 1 small tomato, diced
- 1/4 cup mushrooms, sliced
- 2 tablespoons feta cheese, crumbled
- 1 teaspoon olive oil

Instructions:

1. Heat olive oil in a nonstick skillet over medium heat.
2. Add mushrooms and sauté for 2 minutes, then add spinach and tomato and cook until wilted.
3. Beat eggs in a bowl, then pour over vegetables in the skillet.
4. Cook gently, lifting the edges to allow uncooked egg to flow underneath, until almost set.
5. Sprinkle feta on top, fold omelet, and cook for another minute until cheese softens.
6. Serve immediately.

Avocado Chickpea Toast

Ingredients:

- 1 slice whole grain bread
- 1/2 ripe avocado
- 1/4 cup canned chickpeas, rinsed and mashed
- 1 teaspoon lemon juice
- Freshly ground pepper, to taste

Instructions:

1. Toast the bread to your liking.
2. Mash avocado in a bowl with lemon juice and pepper.
3. Spread mashed chickpeas over toast, then top with the avocado mixture.
4. Serve immediately.

Hearty Lentil Vegetable Stew

Ingredients:

- 1 cup dried brown or green lentils, rinsed
- 1 tablespoon olive oil
- 1 medium onion, diced
- 2 carrots, sliced
- 2 celery stalks, sliced
- 3 cloves garlic, minced
- 1 zucchini, chopped
- 1 can (14.5 oz) diced tomatoes
- 4 cups vegetable broth
- 1 teaspoon dried thyme
- 1 teaspoon dried oregano
- 1 bay leaf
- Salt and pepper, to taste
- 2 cups chopped spinach or kale (optional)

Instructions:

1. Heat the olive oil in a large pot over medium heat. Add the onion, carrots, and celery. Sauté for about 5 minutes, until vegetables begin to soften.
2. Add the garlic and cook for 1 minute more, until fragrant.
3. Stir in the lentils, zucchini, diced tomatoes (with juices), vegetable broth, thyme, oregano, and bay leaf.

4. Bring to a boil, then reduce heat to low. Cover and simmer for 30-35 minutes, or until lentils and vegetables are tender.
5. Remove the bay leaf. If using, stir in the spinach or kale and cook for another 2-3 minutes, until wilted.
6. Season with salt and pepper to taste. Serve hot.

Greek Yogurt Parfait

Ingredients:

- 1 cup Greek yogurt
- 1/3 cup raspberries (fresh or frozen)
- 2 tablespoons walnuts, chopped
- 1 teaspoon chia seeds

Instructions:

1. In a glass or bowl, layer half the yogurt, followed by half the raspberries and walnuts.
2. Repeat layers with remaining yogurt, raspberries, and walnuts.
3. Sprinkle chia seeds on top.
4. Serve chilled or immediately.

Asian-Inspired Tofu Stir-Fry

Ingredients:

- Extra-firm tofu
- Broccoli
- Bell peppers
- Carrots
- Brown rice
- Fresh ginger
- Low-sodium tamari

Instructions:

1. Cook the brown rice according to package instructions.
2. Cut tofu into cubes and pan-fry until golden.
3. Stir-fry broccoli, bell peppers, and carrots with grated ginger until just tender.
4. Add tofu back to the pan and drizzle with tamari. Stir to combine.
5. Serve the stir-fry over brown rice.

Baked Salmon & Quinoa Salad

Ingredients:

- Salmon fillets
- Quinoa
- Arugula
- Cherry tomatoes
- Cucumber
- Vinaigrette

Instructions:

1. Preheat the oven to 400°F (200°C). Bake salmon for 10-15 minutes until cooked through.
2. Cook quinoa according to package instructions; let cool slightly.
3. In a bowl, combine arugula, halved cherry tomatoes, sliced cucumber, and cooked quinoa.
4. Flake the baked salmon and add to the salad.
5. Drizzle with vinaigrette and toss to combine.

Chickpea and Spinach Curry

Ingredients:

- Canned or cooked chickpeas
- Fresh spinach
- Diced tomatoes
- Onion
- Garlic
- Curry spices (such as cumin, coriander, turmeric)
- Brown basmati rice

Instructions:

1. Cook brown basmati rice according to package instructions.
2. In a pan, sauté onion and garlic until fragrant.
3. Add curry spices and cook for 1 minute.
4. Add tomatoes and chickpeas; simmer for 10 minutes.
5. Stir in spinach and cook until wilted.
6. Serve curry over brown basmati rice.

Black Bean Tacos (Lettuce Shells)

Ingredients:

- Black beans
- Shredded cabbage
- Salsa
- Avocado
- Fresh cilantro
- Large lettuce leaves (for shells)

Instructions:

1. Rinse and drain black beans.
2. Fill each lettuce leaf with black beans, cabbage, salsa, and sliced avocado.
3. Top with chopped cilantro.
4. Serve immediately.

Spaghetti Squash Primavera

Ingredients:

- Spaghetti squash
- Zucchini
- Cherry tomatoes
- Fresh basil
- Olive oil
- Grated Parmesan cheese

Instructions:

1. Preheat the oven to 400°F (200°C). Halve spaghetti squash, remove seeds, and bake cut side down for 35-40 minutes.
2. While squash bakes, sauté sliced zucchini and halved cherry tomatoes in olive oil until tender.
3. Scrape cooked spaghetti squash strands into a bowl. Toss with sautéed vegetables and basil.
4. Top with grated Parmesan before serving.

Barley, Roasted Beet & Goat Cheese Salad

Ingredients:

- Pearled barley
- Roasted beets
- Arugula
- Goat cheese
- Walnuts
- Balsamic vinegar

Instructions:

1. Cook barley according to package instructions; let cool.
2. Roast beets, then peel and dice.
3. In a large bowl, combine barley, roasted beets, arugula, crumbled goat cheese, and walnuts.
4. Drizzle with balsamic vinegar and toss gently.

White Bean and Kale Soup

Ingredients:

- Cannellini beans
- Kale
- Carrot
- Celery
- Onion
- Thyme

Instructions:

1. In a large pot, sauté chopped onion, carrot, and celery until softened.
2. Add cannellini beans and enough water or broth to cover.
3. Season with thyme and simmer for 20 minutes.
4. Stir in chopped kale and cook until wilted.
5. Serve hot.

Stuffed Bell Peppers

Ingredients:

- Bell peppers
- Quinoa
- Lean ground turkey or cooked lentils
- Corn
- Black beans
- Ground cumin

Instructions:

1. Preheat the oven to 375°F (190°C). Cut tops off bell peppers and remove seeds.
2. Cook quinoa according to package instructions.
3. In a bowl, combine cooked quinoa, turkey or lentils, corn, black beans, and cumin.
4. Stuff peppers with mixture and place in a baking dish.
5. Bake for 35 minutes, until the peppers are tender.

Overnight Chia Pudding

Ingredients:

- Chia seeds
- Unsweetened almond milk
- Fresh berries
- Vanilla extract

Instructions:

1. In a jar, mix chia seeds with almond milk and a splash of vanilla.
2. Stir well and refrigerate overnight.
3. In the morning, stir again and top with fresh berries before serving.

Roasted Sweet Potato & Spinach Bowl

Ingredients:

- Sweet potato
- Fresh spinach
- Pumpkin seeds
- Chickpeas
- Lemon-tahini dressing

Instructions:

1. Preheat the oven to 400°F (200°C). Cube sweet potato and roast for 30 minutes.
2. Rinse and drain chickpeas.
3. In bowls, layer fresh spinach, roasted sweet potato, and chickpeas.
4. Sprinkle with pumpkin seeds and drizzle with lemon-tahini dressing.

Preparation Steps to Preserve Low GI

Technique is as important as ingredient choice for low-GI cooking:

1. Favor whole, unrefined carbohydrates (steel-cut oats, barley, quinoa) and limit processed versions (instant oats, white rice/bread) as refining increases GI.
2. Cook grains and legumes just until tender. Overcooking can raise GI by breaking down fiber.
3. Pair carbs with protein (beans, eggs, tofu, fish, yogurt) and healthy fats (olive oil, avocado, nuts/seeds) to slow digestion and moderate blood sugar.
4. Keep skins on produce for extra fiber.
5. Prioritize roasting, steaming, and baking; avoid deep-frying, which adds calories and increases GL.
6. Add acid (lemon, vinegar) or spices (cinnamon, turmeric) to slow carb absorption.
7. Use fresh or frozen vegetables for bulk and nutrition frozen works as well as fresh.
8. Replace added sugars with fruit or spice for natural sweetness, keeping GI low.

Follow these steps to retain low-GI characteristics and maximize meal satisfaction.

Customization Framework: Swaps for Any Need

These recipes are easy to modify for dietary preferences:

Protein Swaps:

- Swap beans or lentils for meat in stews, soups, tacos, and salads. Legumes remain low-GI and provide fiber.
- Replace poultry or fish with tofu, tempeh, or more beans for plant-based meals.
- Use chickpea flour omelets instead of eggs for vegan versions.

Plant-Based Variants:

- Substitute cheese or Greek yogurt with unsweetened plant yogurt or nutritional yeast.
- Choose tofu, tempeh, or legumes instead of animal proteins.
- Use aquafaba (chickpea brine) instead of eggs for baking.

Gluten-Free Modifications:

- Use quinoa, brown rice, gluten-free oats, or millet instead of barley, wheat pasta, or bread.
- Substitute almond, chickpea, or oat flour for regular flour in baking, and check all packaged items for gluten-free certification as needed.
- Many dishes (oat bowls, stews, puddings) are naturally gluten-free or need only simple modifications.

Always check GI values of substitution ingredients if in doubt.

Recipe Scaling for Any Household

Adjust recipes to match your household size using the simple guide below. This helps reduce waste, control portions, and keep meals practical.

Table 5: Quick Scaling Guide

Household Size	How to Adjust Recipes	Helpful Tips
Solo	Halve a 2-serving recipe or quarter a 4-serving recipe	Freeze leftovers in single portions for easy future meals
Couple	Use 2-serving recipes as written	Increase ingredients by about 50% if you want leftovers
Family (4–5)	Double 2-serving recipes or use 4-serving recipes	Scale grains, beans, and vegetables as needed for appetite

Scaling Example

Original Lentil Stew (4 servings)

- 1 cup lentils
- 4 cups broth
- 2 carrots

Solo (1 serving):

- ¼ cup lentils
- 1 cup broth
- ½ carrot

Couple (2 servings):

- ½ cup lentils
- 2 cups broth
- 1 carrot

Family (4–5 servings):

- Use full recipe for 4 servings
- Multiply by 1.5 for about 6 servings if extra portions are needed

Seasoning tip:

When scaling up or down, adjust salt, herbs, and spices gradually. Taste as you cook, since seasoning strength can change with batch size.

Miss-Step Alert: Avoid GI-Increasing Errors

Watch for these common errors that can raise a meal's GI:

1. Overcooking grains, pasta, or vegetables over-softening breaks complex carbs into simpler sugars. Keep grains al dente and vegetables tender but firm.
2. Using high-GI stand-ins, like instant oats instead of steel-cut or white rice instead of brown. Double check labels.

3. Adding sugary sauces (ketchup, teriyaki, sweet chili) can sharply increase GI/GL per serving. Use herbs, spices, citrus, and vinegar instead.
4. Baking with refined flour instead of whole grain or nut flours raises GI.
5. Skipping the protein/fat components, which are key to a controlled glycemic response.
6. Portion creep: Overeating low-GI foods increases GL. Use scaling guides, watch portions, and check hunger before seconds.
7. Leaving out fibrous ingredients by omitting beans or peeling vegetables, which reduces fiber and increases GI.

Pause and reassess if you spot these mistakes. Confirm your ingredient choices and portions with the recipe card, and avoid substitutions or shortcuts that may compromise GI status.

Using these recipes streamlines meal planning and supports consistent weight loss. Reference the index cards for nutrition at a glance, follow prep and scaling tips, and customize meals for dietary preferences without sacrificing GI benefits. Eating this way, with careful attention to ingredients, technique, and portions, empowers you to meet weight loss goals with satisfying and energy-stabilizing meals.

Measurement, Tracking, and Adjustment Tools

A successful low-glycemic weight loss journey requires not just good recipes or shopping skills, but structured measurement, consistent tracking, and purposeful adjustment. Without reliable tools, it's easy to lose momentum, miss dietary pitfalls, or get discouraged by slow progress. This chapter offers practical tracking templates and feedback loops for adults committed to clarity and steady improvement as they restructure eating habits, building on glycemic index (GI) and glycemic load (GL) concepts.

Personal GI/GL tracking sheet for meals and snacks

Objective measurement is central to any dietary change. For those focused on GI and GL, a personalized tracking sheet acts as a daily accountability partner and can be either a simple notebook table or a digital spreadsheet. The essential components include:

- Date and meal/snack time

- Description of all foods and drinks
- Estimated GI and portion-based GL for major carbs (using prior chapters' resources)
- Meal composition notes (e.g., protein, fiber, healthy fats)
- Hunger/satiety rating before and after (1=very hungry to 5=very full)
- ***Optional***: notes on mood, energy, or cravings

Such thorough tracking provides a clear, ongoing picture of dietary patterns. Recording foods, estimated GI/GL, and qualitative hunger and satisfaction helps identify links between meal choices and their real-life effects. This visibility is invaluable for troubleshooting and meal adjustments.

For example, if you're constantly hungry within two hours of certain breakfasts, especially those high-GI or low in protein you can experiment with adding fiber or pairing with a healthy fat. Similarly, analyzing snack entries reveals whether between-meal eating is driven by hunger, habit, or cravings, guiding better planning.

Progress Feedback Timeline: Connecting Meal Choices to Weight and Hunger Trends

Simply collecting data isn't enough; the value comes from tying meal choices to outcomes like weight changes and hunger levels. A progress feedback timeline drawn as a calendar, annotated graph, or color-coded table makes this tangible.

To set up an effective timeline:

- Set a baseline with daily or alternate-day weigh-ins at a consistent time for 1–2 weeks.
- Log your daily hunger/satiety averages with your food and GI/GL records.
- Each week, plot a simple chart connecting meal types (e.g., low-GI with high protein breakfasts) to changes in weight and hunger stability.

This highlights correlations: perhaps you lose more weight and feel fewer cravings when you center dinners on legumes and vegetables or find whole grains at lunch to keep you energized and reduce snacking urges. Use color or symbols to mark "best-fit" meals (where weight, hunger, energy improve) and flag those linked to setbacks. Over time, this visual pattern recognition supports precise and effective dietary tweaks.

Symptom Monitoring Log: Recognizing Blood Sugar and Satiety Shifts

Success with low-GI eating hinges on self-awareness of bodily responses both immediate and delayed. A symptom monitoring log, kept with your GI/GL tracker, helps identify blood sugar swings or satiety patterns that might otherwise be missed until they become setbacks.

Track observations such as:

1. Energy spikes or crashes within 1–3 hours of eating ("sleepy," "jittery," "crashed at 3pm")
2. Time until hunger returns after each meal
3. Cravings for certain foods (sweets, carbs)
4. Physical symptoms: shakiness, headaches, lightheadedness, irritability
5. Digestive changes (bloating, unusual fullness)
6. Mood changes relating to meals

Findings like early-afternoon fatigue or mid-morning cravings can be matched against your earlier meal's GI/GL, fiber, and protein content. For instance, if lunch with white rice leads to a 2pm energy slump, substitute a lower-GI grain such as barley or quinoa. Over weeks, the log clarifies which food choices cause improvement or trigger symptoms, guiding actionable adjustments.

Decision Rules for Weekly Meal Adjustment

Effective change requires action, not just tracking. A concise set of weekly decision rules drawn from your logs helps your plan adapt as your body's needs evolve.

Examples include:

1. If breakfast hunger returns within two hours more than three times a week, review breakfast GI/GL and increase protein or fiber.
2. When increasing cravings or sluggish energy arise, check if GI/GL has crept up in snacks or sauces, and swap them for proven low-GI alternatives.
3. If weight loss stalls for two weeks and logs show persistent hunger despite mostly low-GI meals, check total calories and for high-GI foods sneaking back in.
4. If headaches or fatigue are ongoing, ensure you haven't cut carbohydrates or calories too severely; adding back some low-GI whole grains or starchy vegetables may be needed.
5. When recurring "best-fit" meals show better satiety and stable energy, make them core weekly options, modifying as needed for variety.

Build in a weekly review perhaps each Sunday night comparing your feedback timeline and symptom log. **Decide:** *What worked well? What needs changing? Which meals need focus to prevent GI drift from processed foods or convenience eating.*

Short-Term vs. Long-Term Tracking Templates

The right tools distinguish between short-term tweaks and building lasting habits. Short-term tracking targets day-to-day adjustments; long-term tracking monitors trends across months for sustainability.

Short-term tracking (over 1–2 weeks) may include:

- Daily food and beverage logs (with GI/GL, hunger/satiety)
- Symptom monitoring (energy, cravings, mood)
- Morning weight
- Brief context notes (travel, events, illness)
- End-of-week summary (wins, obstacles, lessons learned)

Long-term tracking (over months) should track:

- Weekly/biweekly average weight (to smooth out daily ups and downs)
- Average hunger/satiety scores over time
- Persistent barriers (cravings, stalls, mood)
- "Milestonc" notes (new habits, effective meals, life changes)
- Space for updating target GI/GL ranges as goals shift
- Monthly "GI drift" checks, with reset strategies if GI/GL averages creep up

For example, you may track every meal and symptom carefully for a month, learning that oatmeal with nuts keeps you satisfied far longer than toast and jam. After six weeks, as habits set, shift to weekly reviews logging only new foods, plan deviations, and key data. If progress wavers, temporarily return to detailed logs for troubleshooting.

Troubleshooting and Adjustment—What to Do When Issues Arise

Challenges will surface even with good tracking. Here's how to respond to the most common:

1. ***Persistent hunger or energy dips despite low-GI eating***: Re-examine your logs for protein shortfalls or oversized portions of high-GI foods. Try adding healthy fats like nuts or avocado to meals to slow digestion.
2. ***Weight loss plateau***: Check for portion creep or "hidden" high-GI foods (instant oats, crackers, sweetened dressings). Use your feedback timeline to spot subtle lapses and recalibrate using earlier chapter templates.
3. ***Surging cravings***: Reflect on factors like stress, inadequate sleep, or missed meals. Ensure snacks are low-GI, fibrous, and paired with protein. Review if non-food factors are appearing in your symptom log.
4. ***Loss of motivation to track***: If daily logs become tiresome, use a highlight system: only document new foods, meals that stood out (positively or negatively), and do a weekly recap. For maintenance, this streamlined method is often enough after strong habits are built.

5. ***Overwhelm from GI tracking***: Focus on the fundamentals: swap to whole grains, fill half your plate with vegetables, and combine carbs with protein/fat. Logging these basics captures most of the GI/GL benefit without overcomplication.

These measurement and adjustment tools emphasize progress, not perfection. They help you learn how your unique metabolism responds to various foods, guiding precise, confident dietary changes rather than frustrated guesswork.

Through ongoing use of logs, timelines, and reviews, you deepen your food literacy and resilience reacting less to hunger, cravings, or setbacks and more to objective feedback. This practice helps sustain motivation, ensure nourishment, and keep you on track toward your low-GI health goals, even as you introduce new recipes and strategies along the way. Sustainable weight loss is never linear, but steady feedback and regular adjustment create a flexible, effective path forward.

Troubleshooting Plateaus and Stumbling Blocks

Even with careful planning, everyone faces slowdowns or feels tempted to revert to old eating habits. Plateaus, unknown hunger, cravings, and the lure of high-GI foods at social events can challenge even diligent low-glycemic eaters. This chapter gives you a framework for identifying what's stalling your progress, targeting the causes, and quickly getting back on track.

Plateau Diagnostic Flowchart: Pinpointing GI or Caloric Issues

When weight loss stalls, it's crucial to figure out whether you're experiencing a metabolic slowdown, drifting on GI, or increasing calorie intake. Begin by asking:

- Have my meals been consistently low-GI in the last couple of weeks?
- Are portions creeping up?
- Am I hungrier, craving more, or fatigued?
- Have changes like travel or stress altered my habits?

- Do my symptoms match changes in eating patterns?

Follow this process:

1. If tracking meals, review for hidden high-GI foods (white bread, sauces, crackers), growing portions, or reduced protein/fiber at meals.
2. If cravings or energy dips return, check whether you're pairing carbs with protein or healthy fats, not just eating low-GI carbs alone.
3. If you've logged steady low-GI meals but weight loss has completely halted, check overall calories. Even low-GI diets stall if portions or calorie-dense foods (nuts, oils, cheese) sneak in.
4. If you haven't tracked recently, resume logging for 3–5 days, noting GI content, portion size, and meal timing.
5. Compare this week to past successful weeks, especially if your routine was disrupted by stress or travel.

Low-GI eating can help regulate appetite and blood sugar, but calorie intake still matters. Plateaus often trace back to high-calorie "low-GI" foods or gradual increases in portion size. Other times, "GI creep" introduces moderate/high-GI foods. Review ingredient lists and snack choices carefully to spot these shifts.

Checklist for Assessing Dietary Drift Back to High-GI Habits

Slipping into old patterns happens gradually. This checklist helps you catch where structure has faded:

1. ***Breakfast***: Are you choosing low-GI bases (e.g., steel-cut oats, eggs, Greek yogurt), or have instant oats, bagels, or sweet cereals crept in?
2. ***Lunch/Dinner***: Has white rice, pasta, or refined bread replaced brown rice, barley, or whole grains?
3. ***Snacks***: Are pretzels, granola bars, crackers, or sweets reappearing?
4. ***Drinks***: Are you reaching for soda, sweet coffee, or juice instead of water or unsweetened options?
5. ***Sauces/sides***: Are you using sugary dressings, ketchup, or sweet sauces more often?
6. ***Shopping***: Do your groceries still include mainly whole, unprocessed foods, or convenient, packaged items?
7. ***Dining out***: Are fries, burger buns, or pizza crust your default, rather than salads or grain bowls?
8. ***Portions***: Are you measuring servings as before, or just eyeballing and possibly eating more?

High-GI foods can return without notice, especially during busy or stressful periods. Frequent self-review using this checklist either after each week or a plateau will reveal subtle

"GI drift". Portion size and food frequency accumulate quickly, influencing results.

Meal Satisfaction Troubleshooting Grid: Tackling Hunger, Cravings, and Fatigue

If you feel hungrier, have more cravings, or notice fatigue, something in your food choices likely needs tweaking. Use this grid to identify issues and targeted fixes:

1. **Hungry within 2 hours:**

   Cause: Meals low in protein or fiber; high-GI carbs not balanced.

   Fix: Add lean protein (chicken, eggs, cottage cheese) and/or more fiber (vegetables, legumes).

2. **Afternoon/evening cravings:**

   Cause: Skipped meals, overly low-GI or insufficient prior meals, stress.

   Fix: Eat regular meals/snacks; balance carbs with protein and healthy fat.

3. **Fatigue after meals:**

   Cause: Moderate/high-GI starches without enough volume; too-large portions.

   Fix: Switch to lower-GI grains (quinoa, barley); reduce portions.

4. **Headaches/crashes 1–3 hours post-meal:**

   Cause: Blood sugar spikes/crashes from high-GI loads; lack of protein or fat with carbs.

   Fix: Always add healthy proteins and fats with carbs.

5. **Hunger despite large meals:**

   Cause: Meals high in bulk but low in "staying power" (e.g., air-popped snacks, white rice).

   Fix: Focus on meal quality protein, minimally processed whole grains, beans, fibrous vegetables.

Generally, pairing carbohydrates with sufficient protein, healthy fats, and fiber restores satisfaction and energy while minimizing cravings and blood sugar fluctuations.

Rules for Emergency Food Swaps During Social Events, Travel, or Unplanned Changes

Life rarely goes according to your meal plan. For work functions, travel, or unexpected restaurant trips, follow these emergency rules:

1. **Find the Lowest-GI Option**
   - At restaurants, swap fries or white rice for vegetables, salad, or beans.
   - Choose grilled/baked proteins instead of fried.
   - Request dressings/sauces on the side; use sparingly.

2. **Prioritize Balance Over Perfection**
    - If you must eat moderate-GI foods, always include protein and fiber to reduce blood sugar impact.
    - Add nuts, cheese, or plain yogurt if possible.
3. **Make Strategic Swaps**
    - Airplane/box meals: Discard cookies/chips; double up on protein/fiber items.
    - Buffets: Fill half your plate with raw veggies or lean protein before grains/starches.
    - Hotel breakfasts: Choose eggs and fruit over pastries or pancakes.
4. **Adjust and Compensate**
    - With unavoidable higher-GI meals (e.g., pizza), limit portions (two slices), skip sugary drinks, and add veggies or salad.
    - Plan a lower-GI, higher-fiber next meal rather than restricting excessively.
5. **Hydrate and Move**
    - Drink water to help manage appetite when high-carb options dominate.
    - A short walk after the meal can blunt blood sugar spikes.

Knowing these rules in advance makes it easier to handle social events and travel and keeps you on track without feeling deprived.

"Back-on-Track" Action Plan Template for Resolving Setbacks Quickly

Everyone slips up. The key is a swift, strategic response. Use this plan whenever progress stalls, mistakes happen, or motivation dips:

1. ***Acknowledge and Pinpoint***: Accept setbacks without guilt. Identify if adherence has slipped in GI choices, portion sizes, unplanned meals, or emotional eating.
2. ***Rapid Assessment***: Spend 5 minutes reviewing the past few days logs, symptoms, and energy. Catch high-GI foods, portion inflation, or skipped meals.
3. ***Immediate Micro-Adjustments***: Plan your next two meals with favorite, easy-to-assemble low-GI options, prioritizing protein and vegetables. Prepare simple snacks (cut veggies, yogurt, nuts) to discourage impulse high-GI eating.
4. ***Reinstate Tracking***: Track meals and symptoms for 3–4 days, including food, GI estimate, and hunger levels before/after eating. Note triggers like stress, lack of time, or events.

5. ***Reset Environment***: Remove tempting high-GI foods from sight. Restock at least three ready-to-eat low-GI staples (boiled eggs, greens, beans, apples).
6. ***Social/Travel Contingency***: Before events, eat a small low-GI snack or bring a portable option (nuts, cheese, hummus). Remind yourself of your emergency swaps.
7. ***Review and Recalibrate***: At week's end, check: Is energy up? Cravings down? Did self-tracking expose hidden drift? Celebrate any "wins" (skipping chips, taking a post-meal walk). Recommit to your next week's plan and swap strategies.

A quick return to structured low-GI eating, environment control, and tracking prevents small slips from undoing weeks of progress.

Progress with low-GI eating isn't perfectly steady plateaus, cravings, and obstacles are common. Your greatest tools are objective tracking, weekly checklists, symptom grids, and fast recovery plans.

Sustained low-GI success comes from rapid, conscious course corrections, not perfection. Using structured troubleshooting, self-review, and action templates, you'll transform setbacks into learning experiences and keep progress steady.

You have the tools to handle any plateau or slip. Apply these frameworks to troubleshoot, adjust, and maintain momentum navigating challenges confidently as you continue your low-GI journey.

Conclusion

Building a sustainable low-GI lifestyle is less about adhering to rigid rules every day and more about weaving effective habits into your routines for the long haul. The frameworks and templates within this guide are designed for more than just short-term fixes; they provide a toolkit for lasting change that flexes with your life while keeping you anchored to the principles of low-GI eating.

Central to turning daily habits into enduring results are automation and repeatability. For example, assembling balanced, low-GI plates by pairing lean proteins, high-fiber vegetables, and minimally processed grains enables your meals to consistently support steady blood sugar and satiety. Making this a default rather than a decision saves willpower and time each day.

Preparing low-GI staples or snack packs ahead of time, batch-cooking proteins, or using visual portion guides for grains and starches further cements the habit loop, so healthy choices become automatic rather than exceptional. Simple systems like prepping breakfast oats or always having boiled eggs and beans on hand transform abstract nutrition goals into tangible routines that reinforce themselves over time. These tools help shift focus from temporary restriction to sustainable living.

However, real life seldom follows a script. Balancing dietary ideals with daily realities means accepting trade-offs without guilt. A sustainable low-GI lifestyle is flexible, not flawless. Business trips, social gatherings, or last-minute meals may occasionally introduce moderate- or high-GI foods. The key is context and proportion. Prioritizing low-GI vegetables, whole grains, and proteins for most meals allows space for an occasional treat or unplanned high-GI option.

When flexibility is required, strategic adjustments such as reducing portion size, pairing carbohydrates with protein or fat, or adding extra fiber can blunt blood sugar spikes and keep momentum intact. If dinner out means white rice or bread, enjoy it mindfully and plan a lower-GI, higher-fiber breakfast the next day. This adaptive approach ensures progress continues without breeding frustration or dietary fatigue.

Knowing when and how to recalibrate your low-GI plan comes down to regular self-assessment and practical evaluation criteria. First, monitor outcomes: stable or improving energy, satiety between meals, reduced cravings, and gradual weight progress all signal effective adherence. If hunger, fatigue, or emotional eating return or if weight loss slows review recent food logs, focusing on portion sizes, snack patterns, and the GI and GL of your typical meals. Has convenience crept in, or portion sizes grown unconsciously?

Compare your symptoms and results to the structured feedback tools and grids provided throughout this guide. If you discover dietary drift, apply immediate micro-adjustments: revert to measured portions, refocus on pairing protein and fiber at meals, or swap out high-GI snacks for low-GI vegetables or yogurt.

Finally, set an achievable pace for change, celebrating incremental victories. Low-GI living is not an all-or-nothing project; it is a flexible diet pattern that accommodates life's unpredictability with resilience and skill. The ultimate success metric is not unbroken perfection but a consistent return to core low-GI habits whenever deviations occur. Leveraging the actionable systems, self-review checklists, and swap strategies outlined in this guide will convert individual daily choices into lifelong progress and health.

Embracing these frameworks and criteria planning ahead yet adapting with flexibility you'll create a sustainable low-GI lifestyle that endures far beyond initial motivation, delivering ongoing results, confidence, and well-being for years to come.

FAQs

What is the difference between glycemic index and glycemic load for meal planning?

Glycemic index (GI) ranks carbohydrate foods by how quickly they raise blood glucose compared to pure glucose, using a scale from 0 to 100. Higher values mean faster spikes. This lets you spot foods that help keep blood sugar steady.

Glycemic load (GL) takes this a step further. It multiplies a food's GI by the grams of carbohydrate in a typical serving and divides by 100. This number gives you a more realistic picture of how a serving of that food will affect your blood sugar. For example, a food could have a high GI but a low GL if you eat only a small amount.

For meal planning, use GI to choose foods that limit sugar spikes, and GL to estimate a meal or snack's overall blood sugar impact. Together, these tools help you create balanced, lower-impact meals, especially when combining ingredients.

How quickly can I expect weight changes with a low-GI eating pattern?

Weight loss speed varies by starting weight, past habits, activity, and consistency. Most people notice increased fullness and more stable energy within several days. Low-GI foods release glucose gradually, reducing hunger and cravings, which makes it easier to eat less without feeling deprived.

Some notice modest weight loss in the first week, especially after cutting out high-GI, processed foods. More often, expect gradual, sustainable loss about one to two pounds per week—when pairing low-GI choices with reasonable portions and activity. Early weight changes can also reflect shifts in water or digestion. Focus on building sustainable habits for steady progress.

Are any fruits or sweet snacks compatible with low-GI weight loss?

You do not need to give up all fruit or sweet foods. Many fruits like cherries, grapefruit, pears, apples, plums, peaches, and berries have a low to moderate GI and can be enjoyed in moderation. They provide fiber, vitamins, and natural sweetness that support fullness.

Sweet snacks can fit when made with whole, minimally processed ingredients. Good options include fresh fruit with a handful of nuts, low-fat yogurt with berries and seeds, or homemade energy bites with oats, nut butter, and a little honey or dried fruit. Dried fruits are more concentrated in sugar and have higher GI and GL, so keep portions small and combine with protein or fat to slow absorption. Always read labels, some snacks contain added sugars or high-GI fillers. Portion size is key: both GI and GL depend on the amount you eat.

Can low-GI eating fit gluten-free, vegetarian, or other diets?

Low-GI eating works with many dietary needs. For gluten-free diets, choose naturally gluten-free and low-GI foods such as legumes, non-starchy vegetables, quinoa, buckwheat, and fruits like apples or berries. Avoid gluten-free baked goods made with high-GI flours like rice or potato; try almond or chickpea flour instead. Vegetarians can focus on high-fiber, protein-rich plant foods like lentils, beans, nuts, tofu, and dairy if included. Other preferences, such as dairy-free or vegan, also fit by focusing on whole foods and avoiding added sugars. The main principle is to substitute high-GI, processed foods with lower-GI, whole-food alternatives.

What should I do if I feel low energy or cravings in the first week?

Some people feel low energy or cravings when starting a low-GI diet, especially after eating many refined carbs. This is usually temporary. To help, include enough protein and healthy fats at meals for fullness and stable energy. Avoid skipping meals, low-GI foods cannot prevent hunger if you eat too little overall. Combine carbs with protein or fat, such as apple with nut butter, to slow glucose release.

Stay hydrated, and fill up on non-starchy vegetables for bulk and nutrients. Cravings usually fade after your body adapts. If low energy lasts more than a week, check your food intake, sleep, and activity. Sometimes a small, balanced snack or adjusting meal timing helps.

How do restaurants or packaged foods fit into a low-GI approach?

Eating out or using packaged foods can still fit with low-GI goals. At restaurants, choose dishes based on whole foods, like grilled meats, salads, or bean-based entrees. Ask for sauces and dressings on the side, and swap high-GI sides for vegetables or beans. For packaged foods, look for short ingredient lists with whole grains, legumes, or nuts. Watch for added sugars and avoid products based on high-GI starches. When options are limited, manage portions and combine higher-GI foods with fiber, protein, or fat to reduce blood sugar impact.

Will I need to count calories in addition to tracking GI and GL?

While GI and GL help control blood sugar and cravings, total calorie intake still matters. Low-GI foods support appetite control, but it is possible to eat too many calories, especially with energy-dense foods or large portions. Use mindful portion control and eat to hunger and fullness cues. If weight loss stalls, try tracking calories for a few days to recalibrate. Combining food quality (via GI and GL) with attention to portions and calories gives the best results for sustainable weight loss.

References and Helpful Links

Jenkins, D., Wolever, T., Taylor, R. et al.. (1981). Glycemic index of foods: a physiological basis for carbohydrate exchange. The American Journal of Clinical Nutrition. https://doi.org/10.1093/ajcn/34.3.362

Ludwig, D. (2002). S.. The glycemic index: physiological mechanisms relating to obesity, diabetes, and cardiovascular disease. https://jamanetwork.com/journals/jama/article-abstract/194907

Brand-Miller, J.. (2003). Glycemic Load and Chronic Disease. Nutrition Reviews. https://doi.org/10.1301/nr.2003.may.s49-s55

Augustin, L., Gallus, S., Comini, E. et al.. (2006). Dietary Glycemic Index and Glycemic Load in Relation to Measures of Body Weight. The FASEB Journal. https://doi.org/10.1096/fasebj.20.5.lb88

Roberts, S. (2000). B.. High–glycemic index foods, hunger, and obesity: is there a connection?. https://academic.oup.com/nutritionreviews/article-abstract/58/6/163/1838374

Bornet, F. (2007). R.J.. Glycaemic index concept and metabolic diseases. Retrieved February 5, 2026, from https://www.sciencedirect.com/science/article/pii/S0141813097000664

Atkinson, F., Foster-Powell, K., Brand-Miller, J.. (2008). International Tables of Glycemic Index and Glycemic Load Values: 2008. Diabetes Care. https://doi.org/10.2337/dc08-1239

Jenkins, D., Wolever, T., Taylor, R. et al.. (1981). Glycemic index of foods: a physiological basis for carbohydrate exchange. The American Journal of Clinical Nutrition. https://doi.org/10.1093/ajcn/34.3.362